EVALDO HIPÓLITO DE OLIVEIRA
ILUSKA MARTINS PINHEIRO
TACYANA PIRES DE CARVALHO COSTA

MICOSES:

EVALDO HIPÓLITO DE OLIVEIRA
ILUSKA MARTINS PINHEIRO
TACYANA PIRES DE CARVALHO COSTA

MICOSES:

Surface and Systemic

ScienciaScripts

This book is a translation from the original published under ISBN 978-620-6-76031-3.

Publisher:
Sciencia Scripts
is a trademark of
Dodo Books Indian Ocean Ltd. and OmniScriptum S.R.L publishing group

120 High Road, East Finchley, London, N2 9ED, United Kingdom
Str. Armeneasca 28/1, office 1, Chisinau MD-2012, Republic of Moldova, Europe
Printed at: see last page
ISBN: 978-620-7-63313-5

CHAPTER 1

INTRODUCTION TO MICOLOGY

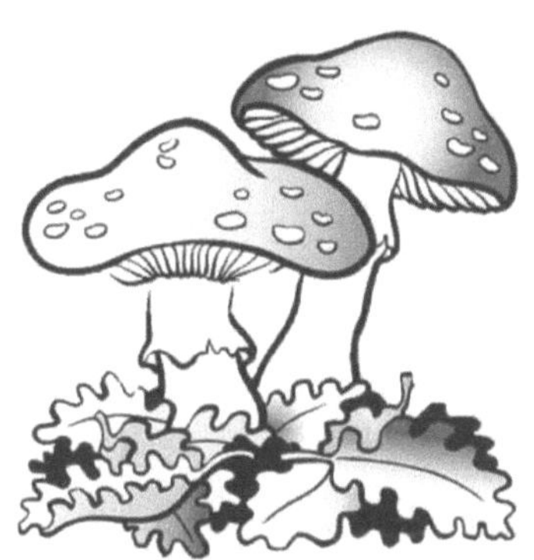

**EVALDO HIPÓLITO DE OLIVEIRA ILUSKA MARTINS PINHEIRO
TACYANA PIRES DE CARVALHO COSTA JANAINA MAIA LIMA
ROSAL**

O For a long time, fungi were considered to be plants and only since 1969 have they been classified in a separate kingdom. Fungi have a number of characteristics that differentiate them from plants: they don't synthesise chlorophyll, they don't have cellulose in their cell walls, except for some aquatic fungi, and they don't store starch as a reserve substance.

The presence of chitinous substances in the wall of most fungal species and their ability to deposit glycogen make them similar to animal cells.

Fungi are eukaryotic living beings with a single nucleus, like yeasts, or multinucleated, like filamentous fungi or moulds. Their cytoplasm contains mitochondria and rough endoplasmic reticulum.

They are heterotrophic and feed on dead organic matter - saprophytic fungi - or live organic matter - parasitic fungi. Their cells live independently and do not come together to form real tissues. The main components of the cell wall are hexoses and hexoamines, which form mannans, ducans and galactans. Some fungi have a wall rich in chitin (N-acetyl glucosamine), others have complex polysaccharides and proteins, with a predominance of cysteine. Fungi of the genus Cryptococcus, such as Cryptococcus neoformans, have a polysaccharide capsule that surrounds the cell wall.

Fungal protoplasts can be obtained by treating their cultures under hypertonic conditions with enzymes of bacterial origin or extracted from the snail Helix pomatia. Fungi are ubiquitous, being found in soil, water, plants, animals, humans and debris in general. The wind acts as an important vehicle for dispersing their propagules and fragments of hyphae.

Fungi can grow in special culture media forming colonies of two types: yeast-like and filamentous. Yeast colonies are pasty or creamy, formed by unicellular microorganisms that fulfil vegetative and reproductive functions. Filamentous colonies can be cottony, velvety or powdery; they are fundamentally made up of multicellular tube-shaped elements called hyphae.

The hyphae can be continuous or cenocytic and tabulate or septate. Fungi from the divisions Ascomycota, Basidiomycota and Deuteromycota have septate hyphae, while those from the divisions Mastigomycota and Zygomycota have cenocytic hyphae.

The set of hyphae is called mycelium. The mycelium that develops inside the substrate, also acting as a support element and absorbing nutrients, is called vegetative mycelium. The mycelium that protrudes from the surface and grows above the growing medium is called aerial mycelium.

When the aerial mycelium differentiates to support the fruiting bodies or propagules, it constitutes the reproductive mycelium. The propagules or organs of dissemination of fungi are classified, according to their origin, into external and internal, sexual and asexual. Although the vegetative mycelium does not specifically have reproductive functions, some fragments of hyphae can detach from the vegetative mycelium and fulfil propagation functions, since fungal cells are autonomous.

These elements are called thalloconidia and comprise blastoconidia, arthroconidia and chlamydoconidia. Blastoconidia, also known as gemmules, are common in yeasts and are derived by budding from the mother cell. Sometimes the blastoconidia remain attached to the mother cell, forming chains, the pseudo-hyphae, the whole of which is the pseudomycelium.

Arthroconidia are formed by fragmentation of the hyphae into rectangular segments. They are found in fungi of the genus Geotrichum, Coccidioides immitis and dermatophytes. Chlamydoconidia have a resistance function, similar to of bacterial spores. These are generally rounded cells with an increased volume and thick, double walls, in which the cytoplasm is concentrated.

Their location in the mycelium can be apical or intercalary. They form in adverse environmental conditions, such as a shortage of nutrients, water and temperatures that are not favourable for fungal development. Other resistance structures include sclerotia or sclerotia, which are hard, parenchymatous corpuscles formed by the set of hyphae and which remain dormant until suitable conditions arise for their germination. They are found in fungal species from the divisions Ascomycota, Basidiomycota and Deuteromycota.

Fungi reproduce in asexual, sexual and parasexual cycles. Asexual reproduction comprises four modes: 1) fragmentation of arthroconidia; 2) fission of somatic cells; 3) budding or twinning of the mother blastoconidia; 4) production of conidia. Conidia represent the most common mode of asexual reproduction; they are produced by transformations of the mycelium's own vegetative system. The cells that give rise to conidia are called conidiogenous cells.

The conidia can be hyaline or pigmented, usually dark - the phaeoconidia; and they can have different shapes - spherical, fusiform, cylindrical, pyriform, etc.; have smooth or rough walls; be formed of a single cell or have septa in one or two planes; and be isolated or grouped together.The hyphae can produce branches, some perpendicular to the mycelium, giving rise to conidiophores, from which conidia are formed. Normally, the conidia originate at the end of the conidiophore, which may or may not be branched. Sometimes, which is not very common, they are born anywhere in the vegetative mycelium, in which case they are called sessile conidia, as in Trichophyton rubrum.

The conidiophore and the conidiogenous cell can form well-differentiated, peculiar structures, the fruiting apparatus, also called conidiation, which allows the identification of some pathogenic fungi. In the aspergillus-type conidiation apparatus, the conidia form chains on phialides, bottle-shaped structures, around a vesicle which is a dilation at the end of the conidiophore.

Penicillium lacks the vesicle at the end of the conidiophores, which branch out, giving them a brush-like appearance. As in aspergillus, the conidia form chains that are distributed over the phialides.

When a filamentous fungus forms conidia of different sizes, the largest is called a macroconidium and the smallest a microconidium. Some fungi form a pyriform fruiting body called a pycnidium, inside which conidiophores develop, with their conidia the pycnidioconidia. This structure is found in Pyrenochaeta romeroi, the agent of eumycetoma.

The internal asexual propagules originate from globose sporangia, by a process of cleavage of their cytoplasm, and are known as sporangiospores or spores. By rupturing the sporangium, the spores are released.

Sexualised spores originate from the fusion of sexually differentiated structures. The haploid nucleus of a donor cell fuses with the haploid nucleus of a recipient cell to form a zygote.

Subsequently, by meiotic division, four or eight haploid nuclei originate, some of which will recombine genetically. The internal sex spores are called ascospores and are formed inside sac-like structures called asci. The asci can be simple, as in yeasts of the genera Saccharomyces and Hansenula, or distributed in locules or cavities of the mycelium, within a stroma, the ascostroma, or even esters contained in fruiting bodies, the ascocarps.

Three types of ascocarps are well known: cleistothecium, perithecium and apothecium. The cleistothecium is a globose, closed structure with a wall formed by closely packed hyphae, with an indeterminate number of asci, each containing eight ascospores. The perithecium is a generally pyriform structure, within which the asci arise from a haemenical layer and are arranged in a palisade, e.g. Leptosphaeria senegalensis, Neotestudina rosatii. The apothecium is an open, cup-shaped ascocarp where the asci are located. Fungi that reproduce by ascospores or basidiospores are perfect fungi. The sexual forms are sporadic and contribute, through genetic recombination, to perfecting the species. In general, these fungi also produce asexual structures, the conidia, which ensure their dissemination. Many fungi in which the sexual form of reproduction has not yet been recognised are included among the imperfect fungi. When the perfect form of a fungus is described, it is given another name. For example, the yeast-like fungus, Cryptococcus neoformans, in its perfect stage is called Filobasidiella neoformans.

The sexual phase of fungi is called teleomorphic and the asexual phase is called anamorphic. Most yeasts reproduce asexually by budding or twinning and by binary fission. In the budding process, the mother cell gives rise to a bud, the blastoconidium, which grows and receives a nucleus after dividing the nucleus of the mother cell. In binary fission, the mother cell divides into two cells of equal size, in a similar way to bacteria. In their evolutionary cycle, some yeasts, such as Saccharomyces cerevisiae, can give rise to sexual spores, ascospores, after two cells experience cell and nuclear fusion, followed by meiosis.

The phenomenon of parasexuality has been demonstrated in Aspergillus. It consists of the fusion of hyphae and the formation of a heterocarion containing haploid nuclei. Sometimes these nuclei fuse and give rise to heterozygous diploid nuclei whose homologous chromosomes undergo recombination during mitosis. Although these recombinants are rare, the parasexual cycle is important in the evolution of some fungi.

Fungi are heterotrophic microorganisms and most of them are obligate aerobes. However, certain fermenting yeasts, which are facultative aerobes, thrive in environments with little or no oxygen.

Fungi can germinate, albeit slowly, in a low-oxygen atmosphere. Vegetative growth and asexual reproduction occur under these conditions, while sexual reproduction only takes place in an oxygen-rich atmosphere. Under aerobic conditions, the hexose monophosphate pathway is responsible for 30 per cent of glycolysis. Under anaerobic conditions, the classic pathway used by most yeasts is the Embden-Meyerhof pathway, which results in the formation of pyruvate.

Some yeasts, such as Saccharomyces cerevisiae, carry out the alcoholic fermentation process of great industrial importance in the manufacture of beverages and in baking.

Fungi produce enzymes such as lipases, invertases, lactases, proteinases, amylases, etc., which hydrolyse the substrate making it assimilable through active and passive transport mechanisms. Some substrates can induce the formation of degradative enzymes; there are fungi that hydrolyse organic substances such as chitin, bone, leather and even plastic materials.

Many fungal species can grow in minimal media containing ammonia or nitrites as nitrogen sources. The preferred organic substances are simple carbohydrates such as D-glucose and mineral salts such as sulphates and phosphates. Trace elements such as iron, zinc, manganese, copper, molybdenum and calcium are required in small quantities. However, some fungi require growth factors, which they are unable to synthesise, in particular vitamins such as thiamine, biotin, riboflavin, pantothenic acid etc.Like all living things, fungi need water to grow. Some are halophilic, growing in an environment with a high salt concentration. Their growth temperature covers a wide range, with psychrophilic, mesophilic and thermophilic species. Fungi of medical importance are generally mesophilic, with an optimum temperature of between 20° and 30°C. Fungi can have different morphologies depending on the nutritional conditions and the temperature at which they grow. The most important morphological variation in medical mycology is dimorphism, which is expressed by mycelial growth between 22° and 28°C and yeast growth between 35°C and 37°C. In general, these forms are reversible. The mycelial (M) or saprophytic phase is the infective form and is present in the soil, on plants. The yeast (L or Y) or parasitic phase is found in tissues. This phenomenon is known as fungal dimorphism and is observed among medically important fungi such as Histoplasma capsulatum, Blastomyces dermatitidis, Paracoccidioides brasiliensis and Sporothrix schenckii. In Candida albicans, the infecting saprophytic form is the yeast-like form and the parasitic form, isolated from tissues, is the mycelial form. In the laboratory, dimorphism can be reproduced through variations in incubation temperature, O2 tension and specific culture media. In this way it was possible to classify as dimorphic fungi in which only one of the forms was known, for example, the agents of chromoblastomycosis. Pleomorphism in dermatophytes is expressed through the loss of reproductive structures or conidia, with morphological variations in the colony. These structures can be recovered in retro-cultures, after inoculation in laboratory animals or in media enriched with soil. Although the most favourable pH for fungal growth is between 5, 6 and 7, most fungi can tolerate wide variations in pH. Filamentous fungi can grow in the range between 1.5 and 11, but yeasts cannot tolerate alkaline pH. The pigmentation of fungi is often related to the pH of the substrate. Media with a pH between 5 and 6, with high sugar concentrations and high osmotic pressure, such as jellies, favour the development of fungi in the portions in contact with air. Fungi grow more slowly than bacteria and their cultures need an average of 7 to 15 days or more of incubation. In order to prevent bacterial growth, which can inhibit or overlap with that of the fungus, broad-spectrum antibacterials such as chloramphenicol should be added to the culture media. Cyclohexamide can also be added to reduce the growth of saprophytic fungi contaminating pathogenic fungal cultures. Many fungal species require light for their development; others are inhibited by it and still others are indifferent to this agent. In general, direct sunlight, due to ultraviolet radiation, is a fungicidal element. Through different processes, fungi can produce various metabolites, such as antibiotics, of which penicillin is the best known, and mycotoxins, such as aflatoxins, which give them selective advantages.

CLASSIFICATION OF FUNGI

The Fungi Kingdom is divided into six phyla or divisions, four of which are of medical importance: Zygomycota, Ascomycota, Basidiomycota and Deuteromycota. Fungi have been used in biotechnology for many years. Aspergillus niger, for example, has been used to produce citric acid for food and drink since 1914. The yeast Saccharomyces cerevisiae is used to make bread and vinegar. These organisms are also used as biological pest control. In 1990, the Entomorphaga fungus proliferated unexpectedly and eliminated the moths that were destroying trees in the eastern United States. In contrast to these beneficial effects, fungi can cause undesirable effects for industry and agriculture due to their nutritional adaptations. As most of us have observed, fungi that spoil fruit, seeds and vegetables are relatively common, but spoilage caused by bacteria is not.

CHAPTER 2

FUNGAL DIAGNOSIS

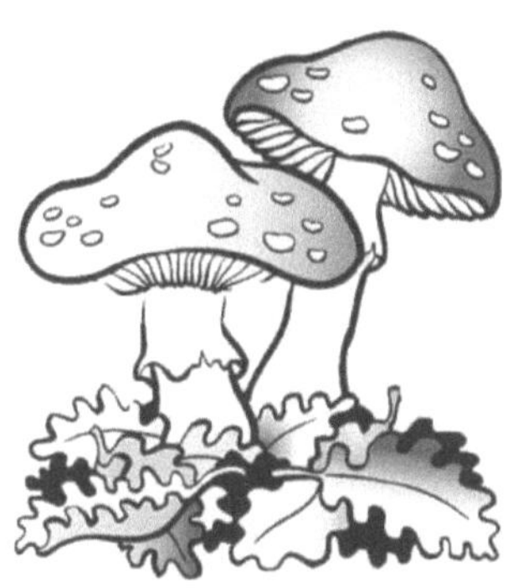

EVALDO HIPÓLITO DE OLIVEIRA ILUSKA MARTINS PINHEIRO TACYANA PIRES DE CARVALHO COSTA JANAINA MAIA LIMA ROSAL

A detailed patient history is essential for the successful laboratory diagnosis of fungal infections. Checking the clinical and epidemiological history and the findings of imaging tests can guide the medical team towards the best diagnostic approach. This data indicates the most appropriate processing for etiological clarification, including the choice of technique for microscopic examination (visualisation of the fungus in its morphology) and the choice of culture medium, temperature and incubation time (isolation of the fungus for later identification). Unfortunately, in most hospitals in Brazil, the collection process, analysis and diagnostic techniques are carried out in separate stages and it is very common for the clinical doctor, pathologist and mycologist/microbiologist to work in isolation to diagnose the disease. Lack of information and/or inconsistency cause delays and failures in diagnosis, leading to longer hospital stays and worsening of the patient's clinical condition.Some fungi have very distinct morphology that is easy to characterise. The ease with which they can grow in culture media is also a characteristic that helps to identify some fungi.

For a successful fungal diagnosis, the type and quality of the biological sample collected and submitted to the mycology laboratory are fundamental factors for the successful isolation and identification of the etiological agent. In addition, basic factors such as asepsis before collection and the quantity of the sample guarantee greater accuracy in the diagnosis. Currently, there are well-defined standards and guidelines for optimising the laboratory diagnosis of fungal infections. These guidelines include pathogen identification, serology, molecular diagnosis and sensitivity tests.

However, recent research has shown that in several countries, including Brazil, there is a lack of standardisation of the recommended tests, as well as poor access to advanced diagnostic tests such as polymerase chain reaction (PCR), mass spectrometry and specific antigens such as galactomannan and beta-D-glucan.

The use of intradermal staining to identify fungi is falling into disuse as it is neither a very sensitive nor a very specific test.

In an organised process, we can better measure the time taken for each stage and make palliative resources available until the report is delivered. The sample processing phase has sub-phases that distinguish the step-by-step process that determines the correct identification of a fungus.

There are fungi that are very difficult to identify at the species level. An example of this is the risk bulletin released in 2017 by Anvisa (National Health Surveillance Agency), where the identification of suspected Candida auris infections

The techniques currently used to identify fungi are:

- Macroscopic observation (direct examination) of the fungus:

Observing the growing fungus can provide several important pieces of information for its identification. However, the culture needs to be pure to avoid errors in the suggestive identification of the fungus.

For filamentous fungi, it is important to check the characteristics of the culture in terms of:

- Texture: cottony, downy, velvety, powdery (furfaceous), sandy or glabrous.

- Relief: cerebriform, rough, apiculate or crateriform.

- Borders: various designs (fringes).

- Pigmentation: obverse and reverse, diffusible or non-diffusible.

- Size: variable (quantity and quality of substrate).

In order to identify yeast-like fungi grown on solid media, the texture, topography, edge and colour of the culture must be observed, and in the case of liquid media, the formation of a film.

DIRECT VISUALISATION OF THE FUNGUS AND HISTOPATHOLOGICAL ANALYSIS BY LIGHT MICROSCOPY

Some fungi have a very distinct morphological appearance and microscopic examination can be very useful. As well as being quick and inexpensive, it provides the doctor with quick information, indicating whether it really is a fungal infection and even delimiting the diagnosis for some genera.

In order to visualise the fungus microscopically, a sufficient quantity of samples must be collected. The collection, transport and storage of the sample must avoid deterioration and cross-contamination of the material. There are various kits on the market that provide needles, swabs and vials that enable these steps to be carried out safely.

In the microbiological laboratory, the collected samples are spread on slides and attempted to be viewed under an optical microscope. In general, most fungal samples do not allow the material to be viewed "fresh", either due to the lack of staining and contrast of the structures or due to the type of sample or dangerousness, and so the spread samples are fixed and stained on microscope slides and viewed under an optical microscope. Depending on the type of sample, the location of the body where it was collected and the clinical suspicion, the technique and/or type of stain to be used on the sample can be defined.

The dyes are classified as acidic or basic and can stain the reproductive and vegetative structures of fungi, helping with their morphological characterisation and subsequent identification. Fungi can be stained with: India ink, Giemsa, Gram (violent crystal, lugol, safranin or fuchsin), Amann's lactophenol with cotton blue, among others.

For the identification of filamentous fungi, microscopic observation of the fungus will be based on the morphological differences of the reproductive structures and the ontogeny of the spores. For the identification of yeast fungi, microscopic characterisation of both the cells in direct preparations and in microcultivation on slides will be based on the observation of: the characteristic of the cell (yeast), the presence of blastospores, pseudohyphae, germ tubes, chlamydospores, arthrospores, asci, ascospores and capsule.

In some situations of suspected alterations or deep infections, it is necessary to collect and examine smears or small tissue sections. The tissue is prepared and micro-cut, fixed on microscopy slides, stained and samples are cultured to identify fungi. Culture is still considered the "gold standard" for diagnosing fungi.

Despite its slow results, it is carried out in practically every laboratory in the world. Even if the fungus has been identified during microscopic visualisation, it is recommended that the sample be placed in a culture medium for fungal growth and identification. The choice of culture medium depends on the clinical information and type of sample received.The first cultivation is usually done on Sabouraud medium. After growth, a sample is analysed to check for aspects of the developing fungus. It may then be necessary to transfer part of the fungus to another specific culture medium with antibiotics and/or dyes. In this way, specific characteristics of the fungus' development can be observed, helping to identify it and test its sensitivity to antifungal drugs. In the case of suspected infection by dimorphic fungi, it is essential to convert the mycelium/leaven forms in order to correctly identify the etiological agent. Examples of dimorphic fungi are Paracoccidioides brasiliensis, Coccidioides immitis, Histoplasma capsulatum, Blastomyces dermatitidis, Candida albicans and others.

BIOCHEMICAL TESTS FOR IDENTIFYING FUNGI

Fungi are heterotrophic beings, meaning that they need to absorb nutrients from the environment, such as carbohydrates, in order to produce energy. Their cells have organelles and function similarly to animal cells, so fungi absorb nutrients, metabolise them and release secondary compounds, enzymes and carbon dioxide.By knowing the metabolic reactions of fungal cells, you can predict reactions specific to a particular genus of fungi and even differentiate species when using various biochemical tests.

Yeasts can be very similar when observed under microscopy and in culture. To identify them, some biochemical tests can be conclusive. Generally, fungi are tested for nitrate assimilation, fermentation of certain carbohydrates, production of enzymes such as urease (zymogram), oxidation reactions with certain compounds such as phenol oxidase, among others.These tests are effective for determining the majority of fungi. However, clinical isolates can show alterations in their gene expression, making identification difficult. In cases where there is doubt about the identification of fungi even after biochemical tests, it is essential to use advanced diagnostic techniques.

SEROLOGICAL TESTS FOR THE DIAGNOSIS OF FUNGI

Serological tests are well standardised for diagnosing fungal infections. There are various types of tests, each with their own advantages and disadvantages. Some methods are already used as a reference in health services to search for specific antigens and antibodies in fungal infections, such as double immunodiffusion (ID), counterimmunoelectrophoresis (CIE), indirect immunofluorescence (IFI), enzyme-linked immunosorbent assay (ELISA) and immunoblot (IB). Of all the serological tests, the most widely used today is ELISA (Enzyme-Linked Immunosorbent Assay), which is very sensitive. Its advantages are that it is cheap, quick and suitable for analysing large numbers of serum samples, making it the preferred test for some public and private screening laboratories. Serological tests associated with the clinic and additional information can be very interesting in confirming diagnoses. In specific cases, such as immunosuppressed patients, there is a wide variation in sensitivity and specificity. Other diagnostic techniques should be used.

There are validation parameters for serological tests, and each technique is planned and developed with these parameters in mind before it goes on the market to be used in the population. They are:

1. Analytical Sensitivity:

Corresponds to the lowest concentration of analyte that the test can detect, generating a positive result (reagent);

2. Analytical Specificity:

Ability of the test to specifically identify a given analyte for which it was developed;

3. Accuracy (Reproducibility)

Degree of agreement between repeated determinations;

4. Accuracy

Degree of agreement between the result of a measurement and the true value (nominal, real, reference)

FUNGAL DIAGNOSIS BY MALDI-TOF MASS SPECTROMETRY

To aid in the accurate diagnosis of various fungi, protocols have been developed for the use of MALDI-TOF mass spectrometry, a methodology that allows the correct genus and species of the aetiological agent to be identified in just 30 minutes. The device receives software with a matrix of data on the molecular structure and behaviour of various microorganisms. Once the device is able to define the exact mass spectrometry phenotype of the mould etiological agent, samples can be prepared and placed in the device for the identification of the etiological agent at genus and species level.Few laboratories in the world have this mass spectrometry equipment for identifying microorganisms. The high cost of the equipment, the need for trained technicians and obtaining phenotypic calibration kits are still factors that hinder its widespread use. Several research groups have been developing and demonstrating the perfection of phenotypic information matrices for microorganisms. For each microorganism, including strains, the structure needs to be calibrated on the device.It is believed that with the advancement and mastery of the ionisation mass spectrometry technique and its variations (matrix-assisted laser desorption) and the determination of more comprehensive protocols, the cost-benefit of using this technique will be very attractive in the coming years.

MOLECULAR DIAGNOSIS BY POLYMERASE CHAIN REACTION (PCR)

Molecular genotyping reactions are highly specific and incomparably better than fungal phenotyping cultures and observations. Many research groups and biotechnology companies have been testing and demonstrating the precise and rapid use of microorganism DNA sequences for genus and species identification.There are already commercial primers for rDNA15 sequences to identify various species of bacteria and fungi. A multiplex PCR reaction can be carried out in around 4 hours, but it is necessary for the DNA of the fungus to be extracted, which adds another 2 hours to the process. With regard to the cost-benefit of the simple or multiplex PCR technique, we observed that the greatest difficulty at the moment is encouraging and changing laboratory routines to implement PCR techniques as a routine in the laboratory diagnosis of microorganisms.

CHAPTER 3

ANTIFUNGALS

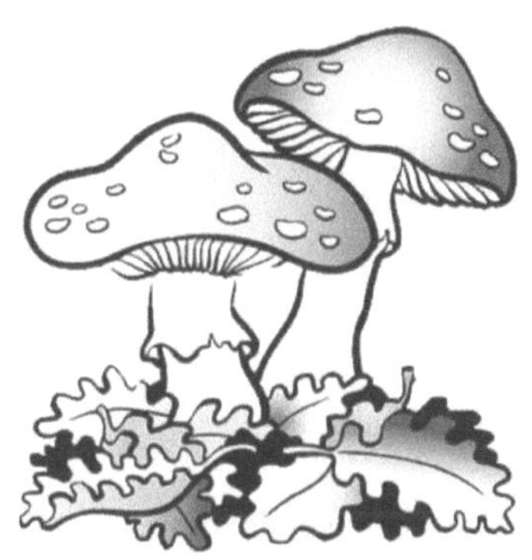

EVALDO HIPÓLITO DE OLIVEIRA ILUSKA MARTINS PINHEIRO TACYANA PIRES DE CARVALHO COSTA JANAINA MAIA LIMA ROSAL

An antifungal or antimycotic is a pharmaceutical fungicidal or fungistatic medication used to treat and prevent mycoses such as athlete's foot, dermatophytosis, candidiasis, systemic infections such as meningitis caused by Cryptococcus spp and others. These drugs are usually obtained through a doctor's prescription, but some are available as over-the-counter medicines.

CLASSES

Polyene antifungals

A polyene is a molecule with several conjugated double bonds. A polyene antifungal is a macrocyclic polyene with a highly hydroxylated region in the ring opposite the conjugated system. This makes polyene antifungals amphiphilic. Polyene agents bind to sterols in the cell membrane of fungi, mainly ergosterol. This changes the transition temperature (Tg) of the membrane, decreasing its fluidity and consequently leaving it in a more crystalline state. Certain contents of the cell, such as ions (K^+, Na^+, H^+, and Cl^-), and small organic molecules flow freely towards the external environment, and this is the primary means of cell death. Animal cells contain cholesterol instead of ergosterol and are much less susceptible to the effects. However, even at therapeutic doses, some amphotericin B molecules, for example, can bind to membrane cholesterol, increasing the risk of cell death. toxicity. Amphotericin B is nephrotoxic when administered intravenously. They are: Amphotericin B, Candicidin, Hamicin, Natamycin, Nystatin and Rimocidin.

Imidazole, triazole and thiazole antifungals

Azole antifungals (with the exception of abafungin) inhibit the enzyme lanosterol 14 α-demethylase, the enzyme needed to convert lanosterol into ergosterol. Depletion of ergosterol in the membrane of fungi leads to structural and functional damage, leading to inhibition of fungal growth.
Azoles block the synthesis of ergosterol, an important component of the fungal cell membrane. They can be given orally to treat chronic mycoses. The first of these oral drugs, ketoconazole, has been superseded by more effective and less toxic triazole derivatives such as fluconazole, itraconazole, voriconazole, posaconazole and isavuconazonium.
Drug interactions can occur with all azoles, but are less likely with fluconazole. The drug interactions mentioned below are not intended to be a complete list; doctors should refer to a specific drug interaction reference before using azole antifungals (see also the Antifungal Drug Interactions Database). Fluconazole is a water-soluble drug and is completely absorbed after an oral dose. Fluconazole is excreted predominantly unchanged in the urine and has a half-life of > 24

hours, making it possible to use a single daily dose. It has high penetration in cerebrospinal fluid (≥ 70% of serum levels) and is especially effective in cryptococcal meningitis and coccidioidomycosis meningitis. It is also one of the first-line drugs for treating candidemia in non-neutropenic patients.

Fluconazole doses range from 200 to 400 mg orally once a day to 800 mg once a day for Candida glabrata infection and coccidioid meningitis. Daily doses ≥ 1,000 mg have been administered and have acceptable toxicity. It is important to note that Pichia kudriavzevii (Candida krusei) is inherently resistant to fluconazole.

Adverse effects that occur most commonly with fluconazole are gastrointestinal discomfort and rash. More serious toxicity is uncommon, but the use of fluconazole has been associated with liver necrosis, Stevens-Johnson syndrome, anaphylaxis and, when taken for long periods of time, alopecia, and congenital anomalies when used beyond the first trimester of pregnancy.

Interactions with other drugs occur less frequently with fluconazole than with other azoles. However, fluconazole sometimes increases serum levels of calcium channel blockers, ciclosporin, rifabutin, phenytoin, tacrolimus and warfarin-type oral anticoagulants. Rifampicin can decrease serum levels of fluconazole.

Itraconazole has become the conventional treatment for lymphocutaneous sporotrichosis, as well as mild or moderately severe histoplasmosis, blastomycosis or paracoccidioidomycosis. It is also effective for chronic pulmonary aspergillosis, coccidioidomycosis and certain types of chromoblastomycosis. Despite its low penetration into the cerebrospinal fluid, itraconazole can be used to treat some types of fungal meningitis, but it is not the drug of choice. Because of its high liposolubility and its binding to proteins, serum levels of itraconazole tend to be low, but tissue levels are generally high. Levels of the drug are insignificant in urine or cerebrospinal fluid. The use of itraconazole decreased as the use of voriconazole and posaconazole increased. The most common adverse effects of itraconazole at doses of up to 400 mg/day are gastrointestinal, but some men have reported erectile dysfunction, and higher doses can cause hypopotassemia, hypertension and peripheral oedema. Other adverse effects reported include allergic rash, hepatitis and hallucinations. The US Food and Drug Administration has made it compulsory to insert a high risk of heart failure warning on the packaging of this drug.

Interactions between drugs and food can be significant. When the capsule form is used, acidic drinks (e.g. soft drinks, acidic fruit juices) or foods (especially calorific foods) improve the absorption of itraconazole from the gastrointestinal tract. However, absorption may be reduced if itraconazole is prescribed over-the-counter medicines used to reduce gastric acidity. Several drugs can decrease serum concentrations of itraconazole, including rifampicin, rifabutin, didanosine, phenytoin and carbamazepine.Itraconazole also inhibits the metabolic breakdown of other drugs, causing elevations in serum levels with potentially serious consequences. Serious, even fatal, cardiac arrhythmias can occur if itraconazole is used with cisapride (not available in the United States) or some antihistamines, such as terfenadine, astemizole and perhaps loratadine. Rhabdomyolysis has been associated with itraconazole-induced elevations in serum cyclosporine or statin levels. Itraconazole can increase the serum concentration of certain drugs (e.g. tacrolimus, warfarin, digoxin). Therapeutic monitoring of these drugs is therefore recommended when they are used concomitantly with itraconazole.

A new formulation of itraconazole (SUBA-itraconazole, meaning Super BioAvailable) has improved bioavailability without the need for an acidic environment in the stomach. SUBA-itraconazole is taken with food and can be used for histoplasmosis, blastomycosis and aspergillosis. Its dosage is different from other forms of itraconazole.Voriconazole is a broad-spectrum drug available in tablet and IV form. It is considered the treatment of choice for Aspergillus infections (aspergillosis) in both immunocompetent and immunocompromised hosts. Voriconazole can also be used for rescue therapy in cases of Scedosporium apiospermum and Fusarium infections. In addition, the drug is effective in Candida oesophagitis and invasive candidiasis, although it is not usually a first-line treatment; it has better activity against a broad spectrum of Candida sps than fluconazole.

Adverse effects that should be monitored include hepatotoxicity, visual disturbances (common), hallucinations and dermatological reactions (e.g. photosensitivity). Voriconazole can prolong the QT interval. There are numerous drug interactions, especially with certain immunosuppressants used after organ transplantation.

The triazole posaconazole is available as an oral suspension, tablet and IV presentation. Delayed-release tablets are the preferred formulation because of their improved oral bioavailability. It is highly active against yeasts and moulds and effectively treats various opportunistic fungal infections, such as those arising from dermatophyte fungi (dark-walled fungi) (e.g. Cladophialophora spp). It is effective against many of the species that cause mucormycosis. Posaconazole can also be used for fungal prophylaxis in neutropenic patients with haematological neoplasms and in bone marrow recipients. The main adverse effects of posaconazole, as with other triazoles, are prolongation of the QT interval and hepatitis. Drug interactions occur with many drugs including rifabutin, rifampicin, statins, various immunosuppressants and barbiturates.

Isavuconazonium is a broad-spectrum triazole for the treatment of aspergillosis and mucormycosis. It is available as an IV presentation as well as an oral capsule. No monitoring of serum levels is required. Adverse effects of isavuconazon are gastrointestinal irritation and hepatitis; the QT interval may decrease. Drug interactions occur with many medicines.

Oteseconazole is a new oral azole antifungal that is used to treat recurrent vulvovaginal candidiasis. Adverse effects of oteseconazole include headache and nausea. Drug interactions occur with rosuvastatin.

Imidazoles:

They are: Bifonazole, Butoconazole, Ketoconazole, Clotrimazole, Econazole, Fenticonazole, Isoconazole, Ketoconazole, Luliconazole, Miconazole, Omoconazole, Oxiconazole, Sertaconazole, Sulconazole, Tioconazole.

Triazoles:

They are: Albaconazole, Efinaconazole, Fluconazole, Isavuconazole, Itraconazole, Posaconazole, Ravuconazole, Terconazole and Voriconazole.

Thiazoles:

Abafungin.

Allylamines

The alinamines inhibit squalene epoxidase, another enzyme necessary for ergosterol synthesis: Amorolfine, Butenafine, Naphthyfine and Terbinafine.

Echinocandins

Echinocandins are water-soluble lipopeptides that inhibit glycan synthesis. They are only available in an IV formulation. The mechanism of action is unique within the antifungal class; echinocandins attack the fungal cell wall, making them attractive because they have no cross-resistance with other drugs and their target is fungal and has no mammalian equivalent. Pharmacological levels in urine and cerebrospinal fluid are not significant.

The echinocandins available in the United States are anidulafungin, caspofungin, micafungin and rezafungin. There is little evidence to suggest that one is better than the other, but anidulafungin seems to have fewer pharmacological interactions than the others.The dose of caspofungin needs to be adjusted in patients with severe liver failure.Anidulafungin is not metabolised by the liver, but is eliminated by slow, spontaneous degradation. No dose adjustment of anidulafungin is required in hepatic insufficiency. These drugs are potentially fungicidal against most Candida species of clinical importance (see Treatment of invasive candidiasis), but are considered fungistatic against Aspergillus. The main adverse effects of echinocandins are hepatitis and exanthema.

Flucytosine, a nucleic acid analogue, is water-soluble and well absorbed after oral administration. Pre-existing or emerging resistance is common, and it is almost always used with another antifungal, usually amphotericin B. Flucytosine combined with amphotericin B is mainly used to treat cryptococcosis, but has also proved valuable in some cases of candidiasis disseminated (including endocarditis). Flucytosine in combination with azole antifungals may be beneficial in the treatment of cryptococcal meningitis and some other mycoses.

The main adverse effects of flucytosine are bone marrow suppression (thrombocytopenia and leucopenia), hepatotoxicity and enterocolitis; the degree of myelosuppression is proportional to serum levels. As flucytosine is eliminated mainly by the kidneys, there is an increase in serum levels if there is nephrotoxicity during concomitant use of amphotericin B, particularly when the latter is used in doses > 0.4 mg/kg/day. Serum flucytosine concentrations should be monitored and the dosage adjusted to maintain levels between 40 and 90 mcg/mL. Complete blood count and renal and hepatic function tests should be performed twice/week. If serum levels are unavailable, therapy should be started at 25 mg/kg, 4 times a day, and decreased if renal function declines.

Echinocandins can be used to treat systemic fungal infections in immunocompromised patients. They disrupt glycan synthesis in the cell wall by inhibiting the enzyme 1,3-β-glycan synthase. Examples: Anidulafungin, Caspofungin and Micafungin. Echinocandins are not well absorbed when administered orally. When administered intravenously, it is able to reach most tissues in sufficient concentration for therapeutic action.

Other drugs used:

Benzoic acid - has antimycotic activities, but needs to be combined with keratolytic agents, as in Whitfield's ointment.

Ciclopirox (ciclopirox olamine) - is a hydroxypyridone antifungal that interferes with active membrane transport, cell membrane integrity and fungal respiratory processes. It is most useful against pityriasis versicolor.

Flucytosine or 5-fluorocytosine - an antimetabolic pyrimidine analogue.

Griseofulvin - binds to polymerised microtubules and inhibits fungal mitosis.

Haloprogyn - discontinued due to the emergence of modern antimycotics with fewer adverse effects.

Tolnaftate - a thiocarbamate antifungal that inhibits fungal squalene epoxidase (mechanism similar to that of allylamines).

Undecylenic acid - an unsaturated fatty acid derived from castor oil; fungistatic, antibacterial and antiviral, inhibits Candida morphogenesis.

Crystal violet - a triarylmethane dye, it has antibacterial, antifungal and anthelmintic activities and has previously been important as a topical antiseptic.

Amphotericin B has been the mainstay of antifungal therapy in severe and invasive mycoses, but other antifungals (e.g. fluconazole, voriconazole, posaconazole and echinocandins) are now considered first-line drugs for many of these infections. Although amphotericin B does not penetrate well into the cerebrospinal fluid, it is still effective against certain mycoses such as cryptococcal meningitis.

The standard formulation, amphotericin B deoxycholate, should always be administered in 5% glucose serum (D/W, dextrose in water), as salts can precipitate the drug. It is often administered over about 2 to 3 hours, although faster infusions, around 20 to 60 minutes, are safe in selected patients. However, faster infusions usually have no advantages.

Many patients experience chills, fever, nausea, vomiting, anorexia, headache and occasionally hypotension during and for several hours after an infusion. Amphotericin B can also cause chemical thrombophlebitis when administered via peripheral veins; central venous access may be preferable. Pre-treatment with paracetamol or non-steroidal anti-inflammatory drugs (NSAIDs) is often used; if these are ineffective, hydrocortisone, 25 to 50 mg, IV or diphenhydramine, 25 mg, IV are sometimes added to the infusion or administered as a separate IV bolus. Hydrocortisone can often be decreased and omitted during prolonged therapy. Intense chills can be relieved or prevented by the use of meperidine, 50 to 75 mg, IV.

Various lipid vehicles reduce the toxicity of amphotericin B (in particular nephrotoxicity and infusion-related symptoms). Two preparations are available: Amphotericin B Lipid Complex and Liposomal Amphotericin B.

Lipid presentations are favoured over conventional amphotericin B because they cause fewer infusion-related symptoms and less nephrotoxicity.

The main adverse effects of amphotericin B are: Nephrotoxicity (most common), Hypopotassaemia, Hypomagnesemia and Bone marrow suppression.

Renal toxicity is the main toxic risk of amphotericin B therapy. Serum creatinine and blood urea nitrogen (BUN) should be monitored before and at regular intervals during treatment: several times/week for the first 2-3 weeks and then 1-4 times/month as clinically indicated.

Amphotericin B is the only nephrotoxic antimicrobial drug that is not appreciably eliminated by the kidneys and does not accumulate as kidney function worsens. However, doses should be reduced and a lipid presentation used if serum creatinine rises to > 2.0 to 2.5 mg/dL (> 177 to 221 micromol/L) or if the blood urea level rises to > 50 mg/dL (> 18 millimole/L). Acute nephrotoxicity can be reduced by IV hydration with saline solution prior to amphotericin B infusion; at least 1 litre of saline solution should be administered before amphotericin B infusion.

Mild to moderate abnormalities in kidney function induced by amphotericin B usually gradually regress after the end of therapy. Permanent damage occurs mainly after prolonged treatment; approximately 75% of patients who have used a total dose > 4 g have persistent renal insufficiency.

Amphotericin B can also attenuate the erythropoietin response and cause anaemia. Hepatotoxicity or other unfavourable effects are uncommon.

CHAPTER 4

YEASTS OF MEDICAL IMPORTANCE

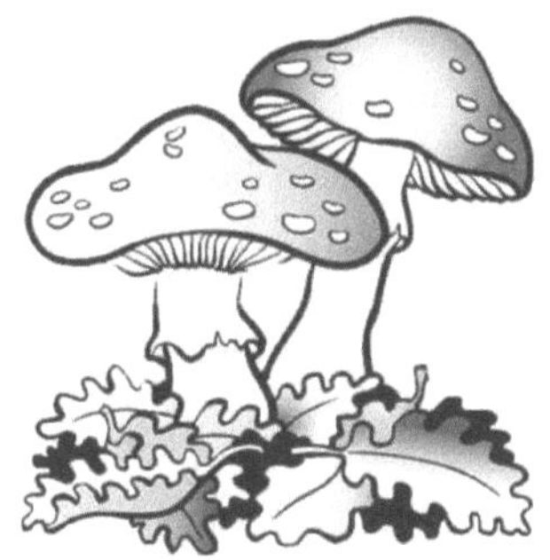

EVALDO HIPÓLITO DE OLIVEIRA ILUSKA MARTINS PINHEIRO TACYANA PIRES DE CARVALHO COSTA JANAINA MAIA LIMA ROSAL

Yeasts are predominantly unicellular fungi within a prophyletic group classified under Asco and Basidiomycetes. They are characteristically spherical or oval and are widely distributed in the environment, just like filamentous fungi, often being found as a white powder covering fruit and leaves. Most yeasts are classified as ascomycetes; they are much larger than bacterial cells and can be distinguished microscopically from bacteria by their size and the presence of internal structures, such as the nucleus. They grow abundantly in habitats where sugars are present, such as fruit, flowers and tree bark. Some species live symbiotically with animals, especially insects, and are pathogenic to animals and humans. Fungi do not have chemical, photosynthetic or autotrophic mechanisms for producing energy or synthesising cellular constituents. They absorb oxygen and release carbon dioxide during their oxidative metabolism. Some fungi can germinate very slowly in a medium with little oxygen. They are capable of facultative anaerobic growth and can utilise oxygen or an organic component as a final electron acceptor, which is of great importance as it allows these fungi to survive in various environments. If there is access to oxygen, yeasts breathe aerobically to metabolise carbohydrates to form carbon dioxide and water; in the absence of oxygen, they ferment the carbohydrates and produce ethanol and carbon dioxide. This

Fermentation is used to make beer, wine and baked goods. Yeasts can be defined as fungi whose predominant reproduction is asexual, the result of budding or fission, and which do not make their sexual states in or on a fruiting body. This distinction has been supported by molecular comparisons, which show that budding and fission yeasts are phylogenetically distinct from each other and from the Euascomycota. An exception is the genus Eremascus, which has non-embedded asci, but the cells are not formed from budding. A similar distinction can be made for yeasts of the phylum Basidiomycota, which are often phylogenetically separated from mushrooms that originate from complex fruiting bodies. In summary, yeasts, whether ascomycetous or basidiomycetous, are generally characterised by budding or fission as the main means of asexual reproduction, and have sexual states that are not included in fruiting bodies.

In budding, the parental cell forms a protuberance (bud) on the outer surface. As the sprout develops, the nucleus of the parental cell divides, and one of the nuclei migrates to the sprout. Cell wall material is then synthesised between the bud and the parental cell, and the bud eventually separates from the parental cell. A yeast cell can produce more than 24 daughter cells per budding. Some yeasts produce buds that do not separate from each other; these buds form a small chain of cells called pseudohyphae.

Yeasts that reproduce by fission, such as Schizosaccharomyces, divide to produce two identical new cells. During binary fission, the parental cells elongate, their nuclei divide, and two daughter cells are produced. Increasing the number of yeast cells in solid medium produces a colony similar to colonies of bacterial origin.Some yeasts carry out sexual reproduction, in which two cells fuse. Inside the fused cell, the zygote, ascospores (in the case of Ascomycetes) are eventually formed. The main yeasts of economic importance belong to the genus Saccharomyces, used in baking and the production of alcoholic beverages. Although the natural habitat of these yeasts is fruit and fruit juices, the commercial yeasts currently used are relatively different from the wild strains, since have been perfected over the years through careful selection and genetic manipulation, making it the first eukaryotic organism to have its genome completely sequenced.

YEAST CLASSIFICATION

Fungal taxonomy has made significant progress based on molecular techniques, mainly PCR and the selection of oligonucleotides with specific probes. The most important pathogenic and opportunistic fungi are distributed in three phyla of the Fungi kingdom: Zygomycota, Basidiomycota, Ascomycota and the Deuteromycetes group.

Several species of the Candida genus exist as commensals on the mucous membranes of most healthy individuals and other warm-blooded animals, where they grow without causing any damage. However, in conditions where the host's defence mechanisms are compromised, yeasts of this genus can become pathogenic.

The main virulence factors of this yeast-like fungus are: adherence, phenotypic variability, toxin production and extracellular enzymes. Adherence is due to the chemical and structural characteristics of the cell wall. The chemical compound that allows adhesion is a nanoprotein, while the structure is a fibrillar cap that covers the wall. Other adhesion molecules have also been described, such as adhesins (lectins and surface glycoproteins), which adhere to protein receptors (laminin, fibronectin and fibrin) present on the cell surface of mucous membranes. This interaction can be influenced by temperature, pH, nutrients, secretory IgA and cell surface hydrophobicity.Phospholipase exoenzymes play an important role in the pathogenesis of opportunistic fungi, as well as an active role in the invasion of host tissue during candidiasis. By cleaving phospholipids, phospholipases destabilise the cell membrane and promote lysis of this membrane. These extracellular phospholipases play a significant role in the pathogenesis of infection and invasion of the mucosal epithelium. In addition, several studies have shown that clinical isolates of C. albicans have a higher level of extracellular phospholipase activity when compared to commensal isolates. Candidemia is among the leading causes of bloodstream infections and is associated with significant mortality. The incidence of candidemia is growing with the increasing complexity of surgical procedures, the existence of patient populations at greater risk of infection and changes in patient demographic characteristics. Its global incidence has risen fivefold in the last ten years and yeasts of the genus Candida are currently between the fourth and sixth most common bloodstream infection in North America and Europe.

However, rates of candidemia can vary geographically. For example, an increasing incidence of candidemia in Iceland was reported in the period between 1980 and 1999, but the same was not observed in Switzerland, where a national surveillance study showed that the incidence of candidemia remained unchanged during the period from 1991 to 2000. Therefore, there are differences between different countries in the epidemiology of candidaemia, highlighting the need for ongoing surveillance to monitor trends in incidence, the distribution of species, and antifungal drug susceptibility profiles. The epidemiology of candidemia has been studied extensively in the United States, Europe and some South American countries.Candida is an important cause of bloodstream infections, causing significant mortality and morbidity in healthcare settings. Globally, among the Candida species isolated, C. albicans is responsible for around 50 per cent of cases of nosocomial infections and the other non-albicans species together account for the other 50 per cent of cases. The non-albicans include C. parapsilosis (28.4%), C. glabrata (9.5%), C. tropicalis (6.6%) and C. krusei (2.6%).

Cryptococcosis is a systemic infection caused by a naturally encapsulated basidiomycete of the genus Cryptococcus. This yeast causes different human infections, ranging from asymptomatic lung colonisation to meningitis and disseminated disease. Cryptococcosis is caused by two species: C. gattii found in tropical and subtropical climates and generally causes disease in immunocompetent hosts while C. neoformans present in urban pigeon faeces, has a worldwide distribution and is a common cause of opportunistic infection.

Specifically, conditions predisposing to a change in cellular immunity have been associated with a significant increase in the risk of getting cryptococcosis, and these include immunosuppressed people due to HIV infections, transplants from organs and receiving immunosuppressive therapy such as chemotherapy. Cryptococcosis, one of the most common opportunistic fungal infections in AIDS patients, is associated with a high mortality rate in this group.

Microscopically, yeasts of the genus Cryptococcus are spherical cells, 4-10 μm in diameter, surrounded by a polysaccharide capsule (the cells can have a diameter of $\geq$ 20 μm if the capsule is included in the measurement), which is an important virulence factor. Cryptococcus neoformans are saprophytes and are rarely reported as human pathogens.

Cryptococcus neoformans are yeasts that are prevalent worldwide and have been identified from various environmental sources, including air, water, soil, pigeon droppings, and foods such as cheese, milk, beans and wine. However, sporadic cases of cryptococcal infections have been reported from immunosuppressed patients, especially those with advanced HIV infection and cancer patients undergoing transplant surgery. The C. laurentii and C. albidus species cause 80 per cent of these infections. However, C. curvatus, C. humicolus and C. uniguttulatus have also been associated with opportunistic infections in humans.

Cryptococcus species can colonise humans via the respiratory and gastrointestinal tracts. The clinical manifestations are generally indistinguishable from those of C. neoformans infections. The most common sites of infection are the bloodstream and central nervous system (CNS), followed by pulmonary sites and the skin, eyes, gastrointestinal tract and peritoneum in patients undergoing outpatient peritoneal dialysis.

Data on the drug resistance of Cryptococcus neoformans is scarce. According to studies, fluconazole and flucytokine have low activity against Cryptococcus neoformans. These authors also found that resistance to fluconazole is more frequent in patients with previous exposure to azoles when compared to patients who have not yet been administered azoles. A study has shown that Cryptococcus species are naturally resistant to echinocandins.

W. anomalus, an ascomycete yeast, is often associated with food and food products, either as a production organism or as a yeast that causes spoilage. They belong to the non-Saccharomyces yeasts of
and contributes to the aroma of the wine by producing volatile compounds. A ability to grow in human and animal food and preserved environments is due to its ability to grow under low pH, high osmotic pressure and low oxygen tension

W. anomalus has also been found in clinical isolates and is considered an opportunistic pathogen in immunosuppressed hosts. Although capable of growing in a wide pH range and high osmotic pressure, it is not particularly tolerant to ethanol and acetate. Several reports have pointed to W. anomalus as the cause of a wide range of invasive infections, the most common being fungemia. It is considered an emerging haematogenous yeast, and there is little data on its susceptibility to antifungal drugs.

On the other hand, the toxins of this yeast have potential as an antimicrobial agent. The yeast can utilise a wide range of nitrogen and phosphorus sources, making it a potential agent for reducing environmental pollution by organic waste from agriculture. The physiology and genetics of this yeast are little known. The first reports on a general physiological and genetic characterisation, as well as molecular genetic manipulation, have recently been published. The new application of W. anomalus is its use as a biological control agent, which is based on its potential to inhibit a variety of fungi in different environments.

Trichosporon is a genus of basidiomycete yeast that produces septate hyphae, arthroconidia, blastoconidia and pseudohyphae. The presence of blastoconidia with hyphae differentiates Trichosporon from Geotrichum. The main species of this genus that lead to invasive fungal infections are T. asahii, T. asteroides, T. cutaneum, T. inkin,
T. mucoides and T. ovoides. Formerly all these species were classified as T. beigelii. Trichosporon species can be found in soil and fresh water, and are part of the normal microbiota of human skin and the gastrointestinal tract.

Infection can be superficial, subcutaneous or systemic. T. ovoides causes white piedra, which is a superficial infection that occurs more commonly in tropical and subtropical regions.

Invasive Trichosporon infection has been increasingly identified over the last 30 years. Most cases occur in patients with haematological patients, particularly those with acute leukaemia. Infection can occur in patients with extensive burns, AIDS and chronic use of corticosteroids, as well as heart valve surgery.

Trichosporum species are the second most common cause of fungemia in patients with haematological malignancies (after Candida species) and are characterised by resistance to amphotericin B and echinocandins. They also have a poor prognosis. Clinical features of disseminated Trichosporum infection include positive blood cultures, renal failure, pulmonary infiltrates, skin lesions and chronic liver disease. Amphotericin B has no fungicidal activity against Trichosporum and in vitro susceptibility to this drug is variable. Flucytosine and echinocandins are ineffective against infections with these yeasts.

Clinical and in vitro studies suggest that azoles, especially voriconazole and posaconazole, are more effective against yeasts of the Trichosporon genus. The T. mucoides, T. inkin and T. ovoides seem to be much more susceptible to fluconazole than T.asahii (T. beigelii) or T. cutaneum. The antifungal voriconazole has very good activity against Trichosporon species, as well as T. beigelii or T. cutaneum. However, the prognosis is poor without recovery of immune function.

The Malassezia genus comprises lipophilic and lipodependent yeasts that are part of the normal microbiota of humans and animals. These yeasts were first described in the 19th century as budding yeasts found on the skin of patients with seborrhoeic dermatitis. It was named after Louis-Charles Malassez, a French scientist, who identified them in the outermost layer of the epidermis of patients with seborrhoeic dermatitis. These yeasts can have yeast or pseudohyphae forms, depending on the culture conditions. In their yeast form, they can be spherical, oval or elongated and reproduce by unipolar budding.

Guého eclassified the yeasts into seven species (M. furfur, M. obtusa, M. globosa, M. slooffiae, M. sympodialis, M. pachydermatis and M. restricta) based on morphology, microscopy, physiology and biological and molecular characteristics. I n addition, in the last decade, seven new taxa isolated from healthy humans and animals with skin lesions have been accepted. M. dermatis, M. japonica, M. yamotoensis, M. nana, M.caprae, M. equina and M. cuniculi. and are now classified as encompassing 14 species. One study investigated the microbiota of rabbit skin and described the species M. cuniculi. The validation of this new species was supported by analysing the D1/D2 regions of the 26 S rRNA gene and the ITS-5.8 S rRNA gene sequences. The results of these studies confirmed the separation of this new species from the Malassezia genus, as well as the presence of Malassezia yeasts on lagomorphs. The development and evolution of pathological conditions associated with species of the Malassezia genus requires predisposing factors in the host. The distribution of new cases is sporadic or associated with nosocomial outbreaks in intensive care unit patients, especially in paediatric settings.

Pathologies associated with infections by species of the Malassezia genus include pityriasis versicolor, pityrosporum folliculitis and systemic infections. In seborrheic dermatitis, atopic dermatitis and other pathological conditions, the pathogenic role of Malassezia spp. is not clearly defined, although their clinical conditions can be aggravated or triggered by this yeast. Malassezia spp. have also been associated with cutaneous and systemic diseases in immunocompromised patients, including folliculitis, seborrhoeic dermatitis, catheter-related fungemia and a variety of deep invasive infections.

According to a case report from Spain, a child who had been admitted to the Intensive Care Unit for 64 days was diagnosed with neonatal sepsis caused by M. furfur. Neonatal sepsis caused by M. furfur has been associated with prematurity, low birth weight and the administration of lipid emulsions via a central line catheter. Treating these patients for long periods of time favours colonisation of the skin, which represents a risk of contamination of the catheter that can favour the entry of the micro-organism, whose growth is fuelled by the ingestion of lipids, thus causing systemic infection.

To facilitate tissue invasion, some microorganisms produce hydrolytic enzymes that destroy the cell membrane and lead to its rupture or dysfunction. The production of phospholipases has been demonstrated by Saccharomyces.

Saccharomyces cerevisiae, the common "baker's" or "fermenter's" yeast, generally colonises the mucous membranes of humans, is part of the normal flora of the gastrointestinal tract, respiratory tract and vagina, but is not usually considered to be pathogenic. In addition, Saccharomyces spp. have been used as nutritional supplements and administered to treat diarrhoea caused by Clostridium difficile.Occasional cases of fungemia in immunosuppressed patients have been reported in older literature, describing three bone marrow transplant recipients in a haematology unit who developed invasive S. cerevisiae infection.Two of these patients died. Genotyping of the invasive and carrier isolates revealed an isolate indistinguishable from that found in patients who were in the same unit during the same period, suggesting cross-infection.

The majority of reports of fungemia are in seriously ill patients, most of whom have had long hospital stays, mainly in ICUs. Almost all of the sick patients had yeast exposure (probiotic, used to treat diarrhoea, or neighbours of other patients treated with probiotics). Most of the patients were immunocompromised, had malignant diseases, received chemotherapy treatments or had undergone complicated abdominal surgery, with the possible mechanisms of contamination being the migration of the yeast through the mucosa via damaged gastrointestinal barriers or lung infections.

In 2003, an outbreak of fungemia caused by S. cerevisiae was reported in an ICU in Madrid. Three patients hospitalised that year were evaluated. Susceptibility tests were carried out using C. parapsilosis and C. Krusei as quality control strains. Krusei. The antifungal agents used were amphotericin B, flucytosine, fluconazole, itraconazole and voriconazole. For amphotericin B, MIC endpoints were defined as the lowest reduction in concentration of the drug exhibiting growth of $\geq$ 90%, compared to that of the growth control. For flucytosine and azoles, the MIC end point was defined as the lowest concentration of the drug exhibiting a 50% reduction in growth.

Rhodotorula spp. are yeasts belonging to the Cryptococcaceae family and are ubiquitous in the environment and in the human body.

They are airborne contaminants that can become commensals on the skin and can be isolated in urine and faeces. In the past, infections were rare; however, today R. mucilaginosa is among the "emerging" agents of infection. Fungemia is more associated with colonised catheters or intravenous solutions contaminated with this yeast. Rhodotorula species have been increasingly recognised as emerging pathogens, particularly in immunocompromised patients. R. mucilaginosa, formerly known as R. rubra, is a urease-positive yeast that is unable to ferment sugars but can assimilate various carbohydrates. Its colonies are characterised by their salmon-pink and coral-red colouring.

Rhodotorula spp. can form biofilm, which may explain the frequent occurrence of catheter-associated fungemia. As with other fungal infections associated with catheters, removing the catheter is often enough to resolve the fungemia.

A study carried out in Madrid, Spain, showed that this yeast plays an important role in hospital infections, especially in haematological patients. The most common haematological disorder diagnosed was acute leukaemia, accounting for 65.5 % of cases. Of the 29 cases of fungemia, 79.3% were caused by R. mucilaginosa, and the majority of cases (58.6%) had simultaneous risk factors. The most common predisposing factors were the presence of a central venous catheter (CVC, 100%) and neutropenia (62.1%). A substantial number of patients (81.5%) received antifungal treatment with amphotericin B. Patients with acute leukaemia had a higher mortality rate (15.7%) than patients with non-Hodgkin's lymphoma (0%), suggesting that patients with acute leukaemia can be managed as high-risk patients and that intensive measures can be taken. Furthermore, it seems that the subgroup of patients without acute leukaemia have a good outcome and can be managed as low-risk patients with a less intensive approach.

Fluconazole is ineffective in vitro for most Rhodotorula spp. isolates, while amphotericin B and flucytosine show good in vitro activity.

Infections caused by Dipodascus capitatus, also known as Geotrichum capitatum, are rare and difficult to treat. Dipodascus capitatus is the teleomorphic stage of Geotrichum capitatum, both yeast-like fungi of the class Endomycetes, division Ascomycota of the kingdom Fungi. This species has already been named T. capitatum and Blastoschizomyces capitatus. This fungus is considered a commensal of the respiratory and digestive tracts of healthy individuals. Opportunistic infections by D. capitatus (G. capitatum) affect immunocompromised patients, however, those with haematological malignancies are the most common victims. Invasive infections occur exclusively in neutropenic patients, particularly those receiving intensive chemotherapy for acute leukaemia. Disseminated infections caused by

G. capitatum are rare, with fewer than 100 cases reported; the use of broad-spectrum antibacterials and the use of catheters contribute to aggravation, manifested by the appearance of lesions on the skin or mucous membranes.

A case was recently reported in Santa Maria, Rio Grande do Sul, of systemic infection caused by Geotrichum in a patient with acute myelocytic leukaemia, with fatal evolution. The 17-year-old patient sought care at the University Hospital of Santa Maria, reporting fever, nausea, sweating, dizziness and pain in the left armpit for a fortnight. Physical examination revealed pallor, fever and crusty lesions suggestive of Herpes simplex on the left thigh. The blood count showed leucocytosis (51,000/mm³) with blastic cells (68%), granulocytes (7.3%) and monocytes (22%); platelets totalled 137,000/mm³ and haemoglobin was 6.1g/dL. The diagnosis of acute myeloid leukaemia with positive CD13 and CD33 immunophenotypes was confirmed. The patient developed sepsis accompanied by haematemesis, melena, haematuria and acute renal failure, requiring peritoneal dialysis. After laboratory tests such as blood culture and microcultivation, genotypic identification was carried out, based on the sequence obtained by amplifying the D1/D2 region, which, when compared with the GenBank database, identified the fungus as Dipodascus capitatus.

CHAPTER 5

FILAMENTOUS ORGANISMS OF MEDICAL IMPORTANCE

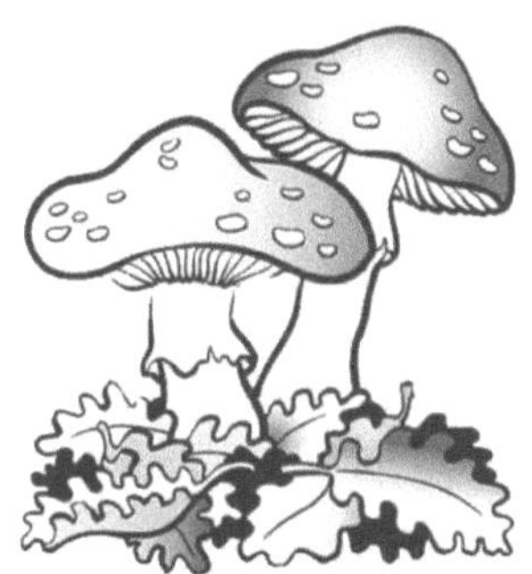

EVALDO HIPÓLITO DE OLIVEIRA ILUSKA MARTINS PINHEIRO TACYANA PIRES DE CARVALHO COSTA JANAINA MAIA LIMA ROSAL

Although invasive infections caused by yeasts of the genus Candida are more common than infections caused by filamentous fungi, the number of deaths caused by the latter is higher. The mortality rate from candidemia in autologous bone marrow transplant recipients, for example, ranges from 8 to 53 %, while disseminated infections caused by filamentous fungi such as Aspergillus spp. and Fusarium spp. can range from 56 to 95 %. The risk factors for developing invasive aspergillosis, or another filamentous fungal infection, have been studied, but despite their incidence and severity there are still few reports on the contemporary epidemiology of these infections.

The characterisation and monitoring of fungi in the internal environments of critical areas of hospitals and of the fungal microbiota on the hands of healthcare professionals, as well as on the colonisation sites of patients, is recognised worldwide as an important measure to substantially reduce morbidity and mortality rates and high hospital costs. In this way, it will be possible to guide appropriate measures for the control of these pathogens, as well as the most appropriate therapy to be instituted within each hospital institution.In addition to the above, fungal infections are of particular interest due to the increase in the occurrence of resistance to the antifungal medications currently available and used in the medical routine. This emphasises the need for continuous vigilance with regard to antifungal sensitivity profiles, not only to avoid cases of acquired resistance, but also to prevent and control these infections. Mycology has developed into a field of science that should demand the attention of all professionals who are involved with hospitalised patients. As reported, fungi currently represent a significant proportion of the pathogens responsible for nosocomial infections, making it crucial to quickly consider the possibility of fungal infection in these patients. It is therefore necessary for healthcare professionals to be aware of the problems that hospital-acquired infections, especially fungal infections, can cause to debilitated patients.

It is important to identify the causative agent of the infection, to understand the types of clinical manifestations that can occur and the environments in which these microorganisms survive, so that patient care can be better planned.

Filamentous fungi are multicellular, with tubular cells called hyphae, of which the whole is called the mycelium. The hyphae can be classified as cenocytic - hollow and multinucleate - or septate - divided by septa or transverse walls. Studies have established the colonies of this type of fungus as being cottony, velvety, powdery, among others, with many types of pigmentation. The dimorphic fungus Histoplasma capsulatum var. capsulatum causes the cosmopolitan systemic mycosis histoplasmosis. Infection occurs as a result of inhaling the fungus, initially focussing on the lungs. In general, in immunocompetent patients, histoplasmosis is uncommon and has a satisfactory evolution in most cases, causing subcutaneous fungemia; however, in immunocompromised patients, such as those who are HIV positive, the infection is said to be disseminated and severe. This disease may represent one of the first manifestations of Acquired Immunodeficiency Syndrome - AIDS. Researchers have confirmed that this disease is a serious problem in immunocompromised individuals, especially those with HIV, and can present serious manifestations that progress rapidly.

Paracoccidioidomycosis, coccidioidomycosis and blastomycosis are also deep-seated mycoses caused by dimorphic fungi.

REFERENCES

ALEXOPOULOS, C. J. ; MIMS, C. W. ; BLACKWELL, M. Introductory Mycology. New York: John Wiley & Sons, Inc., 1996.

ALMEIDA-PAES, R. et al. Immunoglobulins G, M, and A against Sporothrix schenckii exoantigens in patients with sporotrichosis before and during treatment with itraconazole. Clinical and Vaccine Immunology. v. 14, n. 9, p. 1149-1157, 2007.

ALVES, S. B. Entomopathogenic fungi. In. Alves, S.B. Microbial control of insects. Piracicaba: FEALQ, 1998.

ATTLI, S. D. Importance and systematics of filamentous fungi. Campinas: Fundação Tropical de PesquisaTecnológia André Toselloí, 1990.

CRESPO-ERCHIGA, V. ; G"MEZ-MOYANO, E. ; CRESPO, M. La pitiriasis nversicolor and yeasts of the genus Malassezia. Actas Dermo-Sifilogr-ficas. v. 99, n. 10, p. 764-771, 2008.

CRUZ, L. C. H. Mycologia Veterin-ria. Itaguaì: University Press, 1985.

HAMILTON, A. J. Serodiagnosis of histoplasmosis, paracoccidioidomycosis and penicilliosis marneffei: current status and future trends. Medical Mycology. v. 36, n. 6, p. 351-364, 1998.

HIBBETT, D. S. et al. A higher-level phylogenetic classification of the Fungi. Mycological Research. London, v.111, 2007.

KIRK, P. M. et al. (eds). Ainsworth &Bisbyís Dictionary of the Fungi. 9. ed. Wallingford: CABI Publishing, 2001.

LATG..., J. P. Aspergillus fumigatus and aspergillosis. Clinical Microbiology Reviews. v. 12, n. 2, p. 310-350, 1999.

LAZARA, M. S. et al. Cryptococcosis. In: Coura, J.R. Din'mica das doenças infecciosas e parasitrias. Rio de Janeiro: Guanabara Koogan, 2005.

LOPES-BEZERRA, L. M. ; SCHUBACH, A. O. ; COSTA, R. O. Sporothrix schenckii and sporotrichosis. Anais da Academia Brasileira de Ciíncias. v. 78, n.

2, p. 293-308, 2006.

MOORE-LANDECKER, E. Fundamentals of the Fungi. 4. ed., New Jersey: Prentice Hall, Inc., 1996.

PUTZKE, J. ; PUTZKE, M. T. L. The Kingdoms of Fungi. Vol. I. Santa Cruz do Sul: EDUNISC, 1998.

RIPPON,J.Medical Mycology: The pathogenic fungus and the pathogenic actinomycetes. Philadelphia: WB Saunders, 1988.

Mycology

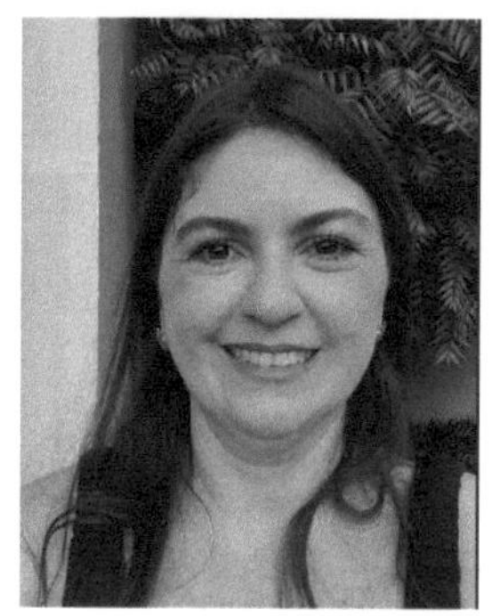

PhD student in Pharmaceutical Sciences at the Federal University of Piauí (2020). Master's in Pharmaceutical Sciences from the Federal University of Piauí (UFPI) 2014. Graduated in Pharmacy from UFPI (2002). Has a Pharmacist-Biochemistry qualification from UFPI (2005). She has a specialisation in Public Health from UFPI (2008) and a specialisation in Microbiology applied to the Clinical Laboratory from IESC (2016). She has experience in Pharmacy, with an emphasis on compounding pharmacy (semi-solid pharmaceutical formulations) and hospital pharmacy (she has worked in the Unit Dose System). She also has teaching experience in Pharmacotechnics I, II and Cosmetology at the Faculdade Integral Diferencial (FACID - 2015). Supervised the Microbiology Laboratory at LACEN-PI (2011-2017). She is currently a Biochemical Pharmacist at the Piauí State Health Department (LACEN-PI), working in the Microbiology Laboratory; she teaches Fundamentals of Pharmacotechnics, Advanced Pharmacotechnics, Cosmetics and Sanitisers, Clinical Microbiology and Microbiological Quality Control of Medicines at UNINASSAU College. He is carrying out research into topical pharmaceutical formulations for the treatment of cutaneous leishmaniasis with a team from UFPI under the guidance of Prof Dr André Luís Menezes Carvalho.

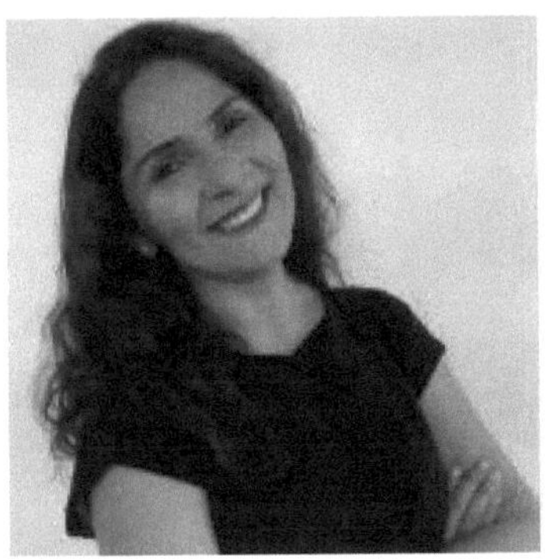

Graduated in Biomedicine from Faculdade Aliança, Graduated in Pharmacy from Faculdade Mauricio de Nassau. PhD in Biomedical Engineering from the University of Brazil with research into the tolerance of fungi to UV-B radiation and heat. Master's in Clinical Pharmacology from the Federal University of Ceará with research into genetic toxicology. Specialised in Parasite Biology at the Federal Institute of Piauí. Contributed to research at the Piauí Central Public Health Laboratory. Lecturer in the area of Health, working mainly in the disciplines of Clinical Biochemistry, Medical Microbiology (Bacteriology, Virology, Mycology and Parasitology) and Collective Health.

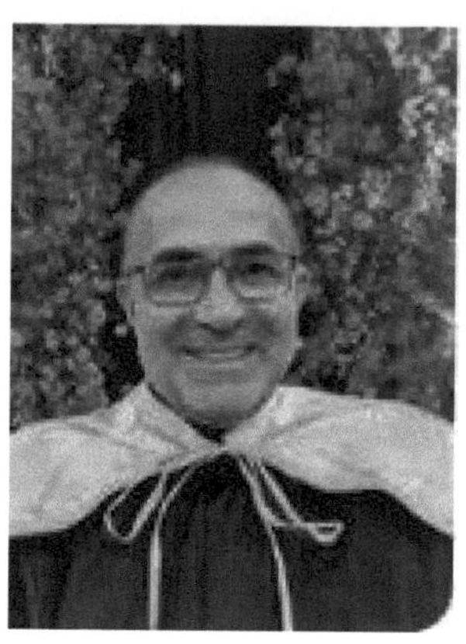

He has a degree in Pharmacy from the Federal University of Paraíba (1990), a degree in Pharmacy and Biochemistry from the Federal University of Paraíba (1991), a degree in Law from the Federal University of Piauí (1999), a PhD in Biology of Infectious and Parasitic Agents (2010), a master's degree in Administration from the Federal University of Paraíba (2002), specialisation in Sanitary and Epidemiological Surveillance (1997) and Clinical Cytology (2005). He was Director of the Central Public Health Laboratory of the State of Piauí-LACEN-PI (2003 to 2007).He is currently an Associate Professor of Clinical Microbiology and Clinical Immunology at the Federal University of Piauí (1994). He has experience in Pharmacy (Interdisciplinary), working mainly on the following subjects: clinical analyses (bacteriology, virology, immunology, cytology and haematology) and Human T-cell Lymphotropic Virus-1/2-HTLV- 1/2, HIV, HBV and HCV (Epidemiology, Immunology and Molecular Analysis). ORCID: https://orcid.org/0000-0003-4180-012X

INDEX

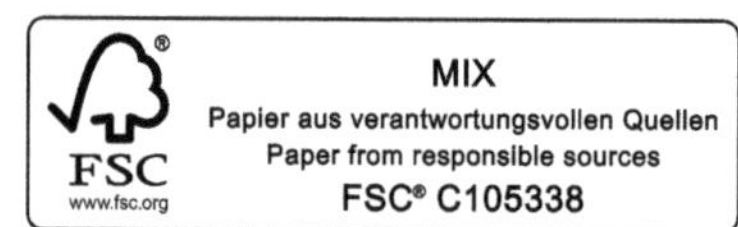

Printed by Books on Demand GmbH, Norderstedt / Germany